WEIGHTED DOWN

WHEN BEING OVERWEIGHT MAKES YOU SICK

OBESITY & KIDS

WEIGHTED DOWN

WHEN BEING OVERWEIGHT MAKES YOU SICK

BY HELEN THOMPSON

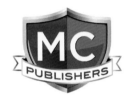

Mason Crest Publishers

MASON CREST PUBLISHERS INC.
370 Reed Road
Broomall, Pennsylvania 19008
(866)MCP-BOOK (toll free)
www.masoncrest.com

First Printing
9 8 7 6 5 4 3 2 1

Library of Congress Cataloging-in-Publication Data

Thompson, Helen, 1957–
 Weighted down : when being overweight makes you sick / by Helen Thompson.
     p. cm.
 Includes index.
 ISBN 978-1-4222-1708-5 (hardcover)   ISBN 978-1-4222-1705-4 (hardcover series)
 ISBN 978-1-4222-1896-9 (pbk.)   ISBN 978-1-4222-1893-8 (pbk series)
 1. Obesity in children—Juvenile literature. 2. Obesity—Complications—Juvenile literature. I. Title.
 RJ399.C6T56 2010
 618.92'398—dc22
                              2010022266
Design by MK Bassett-Harvey and Wendy Arakawa.
Produced by Harding House Publishing Service, Inc.
www.hardinghousepages.com
Cover design by Torque Advertising and Design.
Printed in USA by Bang Printing.

The creators of this book have made every effort to provide accurate information, but it should not be used as a substitute for the help and services of trained professionals.

CONTENTS

INTRODUCTION
FOR THE TEACHERS

We as a society often reserve our harshest criticism for those conditions we understand the least. Such is the case for obesity. Obesity is a chronic and often-fatal disease that accounts for 400,000 deaths each year. It is second only to smoking as a cause of premature death in the United States. People suffering from obesity need understanding, support, and medical assistance. Yet what they often receive is scorn.

Today, children are the fastest growing segment of the obese population in the United States. This constitutes a public health crisis of enormous proportions. Living with childhood obesity affects self-esteem, which down the road can affect employment and attainment of higher education. But childhood obesity is much more than a social stigma. It has serious health consequences.

Childhood obesity increases the risk for poor health in adulthood—but also even during childhood. Depression, diabetes, asthma, gallstones, orthopedic diseases, and other obesity-related conditions are all on the rise in children. Recent estimates suggest that 30 to 50 percent of children born in 2000 will develop type 2 diabetes mellitus, a leading cause of preventable blindness, kidney failure, heart disease, stroke, and amputations. Obesity is undoubtedly the most pressing nutritional disorder among young people today.

If we are to reverse obesity's current trend, there must be family, community, and national objectives promoting healthy eating and exercise. As a nation, we must demand broad-based public-health initiatives to limit TV watching, curtail junk food advertising toward children, and promote physical activity. More than rhetoric, these need to be our rallying cry. Anything short of this will eventually fail, and within our lifetime obesity will become the leading cause of death in the United States if not in the world. This series is an excellent first step in battling the obesity crisis by educating young children about the risks, the realities, and what they can do to build healthy lifestyles right now.

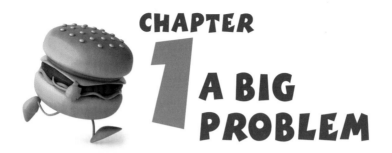

CHAPTER 1
A BIG PROBLEM

Did you know that people all over the globe are getting fatter? There are more than a billion adults around the world who are **overweight**. At least 300 million of them are **obese**.

But it's not just grownups who are overweight and obese. More and more children are overweight too, even very young children. Around the world, at least 42 million children who are younger than five are overweight. In the United States, 15 percent of all children between the ages of six and eleven are overweight. That means that if you had 100 children in a room, chances are 15 of them would be overweight. And if you were to put 100 kids who were between the ages of twelve and nineteen all in one room, you'd be likely to find that 18 of them (18 percent) would be overweight. Then, if you put 100 grownups together,

If you're overweight, you're not alone—lots of kids around the world have this problem, as well as millions of adults.

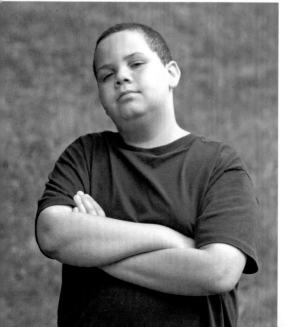

67 of them would be overweight or obese. That's more than two-thirds of all grownups!

WHAT CAUSES OBESITY?

You've probably heard people talk about calories. Sometimes it may sound as though calories are bad things. After all, commercials are always making low-calorie foods sound as though they're healthier, and people who are on a diet will often count calories. It's true that too many calories can make us fat—but we also need calories.

Calories are a way to measure what's in the food we eat. We use inches and feet (or centimeters and meters) to measure how long or tall something is; we use pints and quarts (or liters) to measure liquids like milk and soda —and we use calories to measure how much **energy** is in a certain food.

Each one of us needs a certain amount of calories every day to be healthy and have

What's the difference between being overweight and being obese? Both words mean that a person has too much body fat, so much so that it's a health risk. But a person who is obese has much more fat than a person who is overweight, and the health risks are greater as well.

What is energy? Energy is the ability to be active, the power it takes to move your body.

the energy we need for all the things we do in a day. Even sitting still takes a certain number of calories, but the more active we are, the more calories we need. People who are bigger, more active, or who are growing usually need more calories than smaller people, people who don't move around very much, and people who aren't growing.

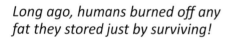

Long ago, humans burned off any fat they stored just by surviving!

When we eat more calories than we need, our bodies store the extra energy as fat. Long ago, our ancestors went through times when they had plenty of food, followed by times when food was scarcer. Their bodies' stores of fat helped them get through the times when they had less food. Today, though, many times our bodies just keep storing more and more fat that never needs to be used. When that happens, we end up being overweight or obese.

To get rid of these extra stores of fat, we need to do one of two things: take in fewer calories, forcing our bodies to use up the stored energy in our fat—or use up more calories by exercising more, which will also make our bodies use up the fat we've stored.

HOW DO YOU KNOW IF YOU'RE OVERWEIGHT?

Experts have figured out a way to help you know if you are in the healthy weight range for your height. It's called the body mass index or BMI. The BMI formula uses height and weight to come up with a BMI number. Though the formula is the same for adults and children, figuring out what the BMI number means is a little more complicated for kids. For children, BMI is plotted on a growth chart that tells whether a child is underweight, healthy weight, overweight, or obese. Different BMI charts are used for boys and girls who are younger than twenty, because the amount of body fat differs between boys and girls. Also, the amount of body fat that is healthy is different, depending on whether you're a toddler or a teenager.

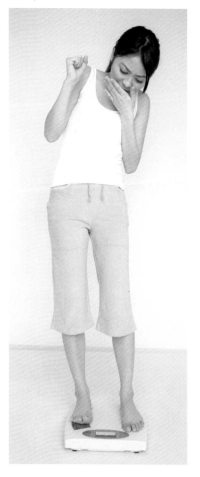

Stepping on the scales can't really tell you if you're over-weight. Use the BMI chart to see if you're too heavy, too thin, or just right—and then ask your doctor.

Each BMI chart is divided into percentiles. A child whose BMI is equal to or greater than the 5th percentile and less than the 85th percentile is considered a healthy weight for his or her age. A child at or above the 85th percentile but less than the 95th percentile for age is considered overweight. A child at or above the 95th percentile is considered obese. A child below the 5th percentile is considered underweight.

If you know how much you weigh and how tall you are, you can look at these charts and see for yourself whether you are overweight or obese—but it's also a good idea to talk to your doctor (even if that seems embarrassing). BMI is not always right, so a doctor will be better able to tell you if your weight is healthy or not.

Even though doctors use BMI to determine if you're over-weight or obese, BMI is sometimes wrong. That's because different types of body tissues weigh different amounts. Muscle, for example, weighs eight or nine times as much as fat. This means that a small amount of muscle will be as heavy, or heavier, than a larger amount of fat.

Imagine two children who are the same height. One weighs 100 pounds. The other weighs 85 pounds. Judging by weight alone, you might think that the 85-pound child is healthier and has less fat than the 100-pound child. If the 100-pound kid, however, is very muscular, and the 85-pound kid has practically no muscles at all, then you'd be wrong. The 85-pound child could actually be both lighter and "fatter" than the muscular 100-pound kid.

2 to 20 years: Boys
Body mass index-for-age percentiles

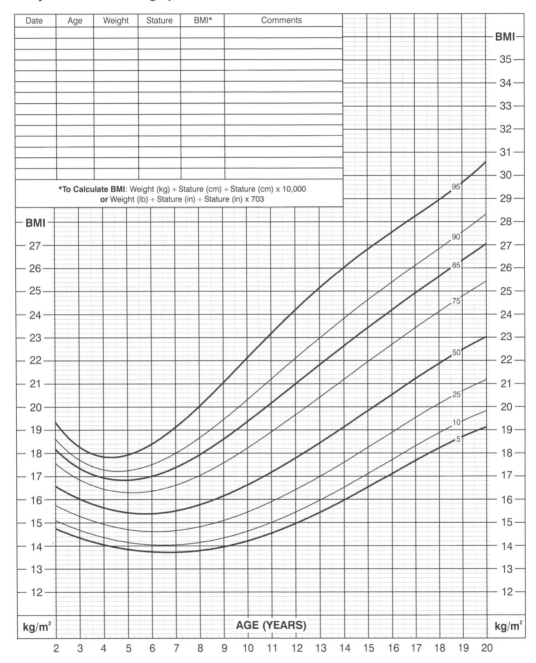

BMI growth chart for boys ages 2–20.

2 to 20 years: Girls
Body mass index-for-age percentiles

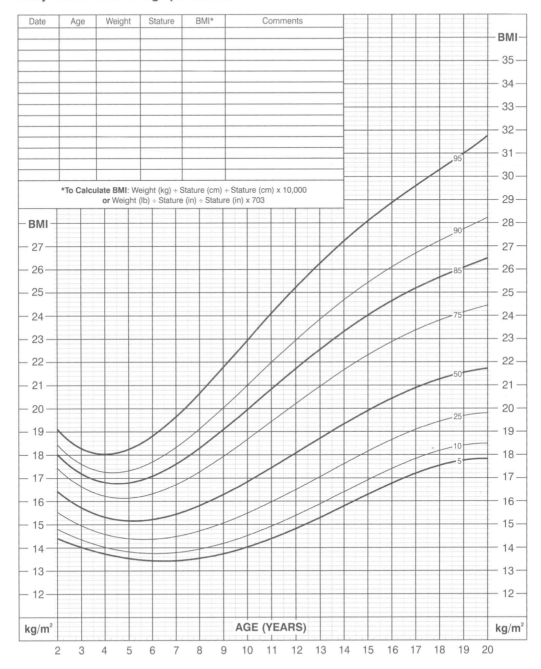

Date	Age	Weight	Stature	BMI*	Comments

*To Calculate BMI: Weight (kg) ÷ Stature (cm) ÷ Stature (cm) x 10,000
or Weight (lb) ÷ Stature (in) ÷ Stature (in) x 703

BMI growth chart for girls ages 2–20.

A HEALTH PROBLEM

Our world is full of messages telling us we need to be thin to be pretty or good-looking. Everywhere we turn—on television, in ads, on magazine covers—we run into this message. Every year, thousands and thousands of people—including kids—go on diets. They buy exercise equipment and join gyms. They drink diet sodas and eat special low-fat foods. And yet people around the world are still getting fatter.

Not everyone understands that obesity is a health problem rather than an appearance problem. Sometimes people think that others who are overweight are lazy or greedy. They think that if those people wanted to lose weight bad enough, they could easily become thinner. Sometimes people don't want to get to know others simply because they're overweight or obese. They assume that people with more fat are not as interesting, not as smart, or sim-

DID YOU KNOW?

A stereotype is a picture we have in our heads about a group of people. It's not necessarily true. In fact, it seldom is, because people are individuals, and each person within a group is different. But many people have a stereotype in their heads when they think about people who are overweight and obese. They think that they're lazy, weak, and sad. They may think people who are overweight are not as clean or that they smell bad. They often think people who are overweight and obese are not as smart and not as likeable as other people.

And that's not true.

ply not as important. They're **prejudiced** against people who are overweight.

People come in all different sizes and shapes — and no one should ever be insulted or treated with less respect because of their weight. People who are overweight or obese can still be smart and pretty and funny. And losing weight isn't easy.

But being overweight or obese isn't healthy. It puts you at risk for getting sick, both now, when you're still a kid, and later, when you grow up. It's a big problem!

What does prejudiced mean? Prejudiced is the word we use when someone thinks differently about others because of their race, their religion, or the way they look. Most of us know that this is wrong—but many people think it's okay to think about people differently because they are overweight or obese. This is a form of prejudice too. And yet we hear fat jokes at school all the time. Grownups tell fat jokes too. People on television do as well. Most of the time, people forget how cruel this is, or how it makes others feel.

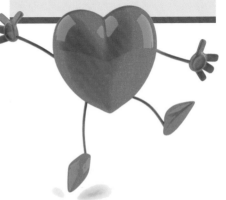

2 RIGHT NOW

People who are overweight or obese have more fat than their bodies were meant to carry. Imagine carrying a ten-pound bag of sand with you wherever you went. You'd get tired more quickly than you would if you weren't carrying that weight. Now imagine that bag of sand weighs twenty pounds— or even fifty. Carrying around more weight than you were made to carry is hard work. It makes you tired, and after a while, it's hard on your body. Adults who are overweight and obese get sick more often, but so do children.

Children who are overweight may get diseases that only adults usually get.

DIABETES

One of the diseases that children who are overweight or obese are more likely to get is diabetes. Diabetes is a disease that affects how your body uses glucose, a type of sugar your body uses for fuel. Like a car that needs gasoline to run, you need glucose to play and study, think and talk.

Normally, when you eat, glucose from the food goes into your bloodstream. Your **pancreas** makes a **hormone** called insulin that helps the glucose get to your body's **cells**. Insulin is like the key that opens the doors to all the cells in your body, from head to toe. When that happens, your body gets the fuel—the energy—it needs to do all the things it does.

What is your pancreas? It's a long, flat gland in your stomach that helps your body break down the food you eat so that your body can use it. Your pancreas also makes insulin.

What is a hormone? A hormone is a chemical produced by cells in one part of your body that acts as a messenger to tell another part of your body to do a certain thing, like digest food or grow taller. Your body makes many, many different kinds of hormones.

What are cells? Cells are the very small parts of all living things, including the human body. You have billions of cells in your body!

But if someone has diabetes, the pancreas either can't make insulin or the insulin doesn't work in the body the way it should. If the glucose can't get into the cells, there will be too much glucose (sugar) in the blood. Too much sugar in their blood makes people sick.

There are two kinds of diabetes—type 1 and type 2. With type 1 diabetes, the pancreas doesn't make insulin. This means that glucose can't get into the body's cells, where it's needed for fuel, and it makes the blood sugar level very high. With type 2 diabetes, on the other hand, the pancreas can still make insulin, but the insulin doesn't do its job very well. The glucose doesn't get into the cells, and instead it builds up in the blood. The pancreas makes even more insulin, but eventually it gets worn out from working so hard.

DID YOU KNOW?

Scientists think that diabetes is probably passed down through families. Kids with family members who have type 2 diabetes also get it more often. Also, kids from Native American, African American, Hispanic/Latino, or Asian/Pacific Island backgrounds are more likely to get type 2 diabetes. Children who are older than 10 are more likely to get type 2 diabetes than younger kids.

Most people who have type 2 diabetes are overweight. It used to be that mainly adults got type 2 diabetes, but today, more kids are getting this disease. That's because more kids are overweight or obese. Sometimes, if kids eat healthy foods, exercise, and lose weight, they may be able to get their blood sugar levels into a healthier range. If that happens, their doctors may decide they don't have to take medicine for diabetes anymore.

OTHER DISEASES

Children who are overweight or obese are also more likely to get many other diseases besides diabetes.

BLOUNT'S DISEASE

Carrying extra weight that your bones weren't meant to carry can cause this disease. It can make the bones in your lower legs—your shins—curve, so that you have bowed legs.

ARTHRITIS

This is a disease you may connect with your grandparents—but being too heavy can cause it even in children. Carrying extra weight puts wear-and-tear on your joints, making them become swollen, stiff, and sore.

DID YOU KNOW?

Some kids can have type 2 diabetes without knowing it. Some of the signs aren't easy to spot, and they can take a long time to develop. And some kids don't have any symptoms at all. The first symptoms of diabetes are usually:

· feeling tired a lot, because your body can't get the fuel it needs.
· going to the bathroom a lot, because your body is trying to get rid of the extra blood sugar by passing it out of the body in urine (pee).
· feeling thirsty a lot, because your body is trying to make up for all the pee its been losing.

SLIPPED CAPITAL FEMORAL EPIPHYSES (SCFE)

These big words mean that inside the hip joint, the "ball" of the thigh bone moves off from the neck of the hip bone, like a scoop of ice cream slipping off the top of a cone. When this happens, the hip joint becomes sore and stiff. Young people who are obese have a greater chance of this happening. SCFE requires immediate attention and an operation to prevent further damage to the joint.

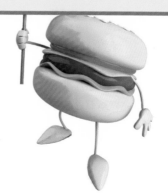

DID YOU KNOW?

Kids with type 2 diabetes need to:

- follow a healthy eating plan so they can keep blood sugar levels under control and grow normally.
- exercise regularly.
- take insulin in pills or shots, or take medicines that help insulin work better in their bodies.
- check their blood sugar levels by testing their blood every day.
- get treatment for other health problems that can happen more often in people with type 2 diabetes, like high blood pressure.
- have regular checkups with doctors so they can stay healthy and get treatment for any diabetes problems.

ASTHMA

Being overweight can give a young person breathing problems. Because it's harder for him to breathe in the oxygen he needs, he may have a hard time keeping up with friends, playing sports, or just walking from class to class. This can create a vicious circle for kids like this—exercising is hard for them because their lungs can't get enough oxygen, so they don't exercise as much, which makes them more likely to gain more weight, which makes their asthma even worse!

SLEEP APNEA

If a person has sleep apnea, every now and then she'll stop breathing for a few seconds while she's sleeping. It's a serious problem for many kids and adults who are overweight. It can interrupt their sleep and leave them feeling tired. They may be too tired the next day to concentrate and learn. Sleep apnea can also be hard on the heart and lead to heart disorders.

HIGH BLOOD PRESSURE

This is another condition you might connect with older people, but more and more chil-dren are getting high blood pressure these days because they're obese. Being overweight means your heart has to pump your blood harder to get it to all the parts of your body. This means the blood vessels in your body have to carry blood that's moving under greater pres-sure. Imagine a garden hose

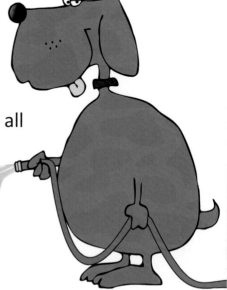

where the water comes out very fast and hard when you turn it on. That's what it's like inside the arteries of someone who has high blood pressure. If the problem lasts for a long time, the heart and arteries may get worn out and no longer work as well as they should. Have you ever seen the side of a garden hose bulge out from the water pressure inside it? This happens when the hose starts to wear out. If this happens inside a blood vessel, it can cause a stroke, a condition where a person's brain doesn't get enough blood.

HIGH CHOLESTEROL

Long before they look or act sick, children who are overweight or obese may have too much of a certain kind of fat called cholesterol in their blood. Cholesterol can build up inside blood vessels, causing high blood pressure, and eventually, when a person is older, he may be more likely to have a stroke or heart attack.

Being overweight can cause even kids to get high blood pressure.

GALLSTONES

When cholesterol builds up inside your **gallbladder**, it can form hard lumps, called gallstones. These can be as tiny as a grain of stand or as big as a golf ball. The bigger they are the more they hurt. They can press on other parts of your body and keep your organs from being able to do their jobs. When that happens, you may need to have an operation to have them removed.

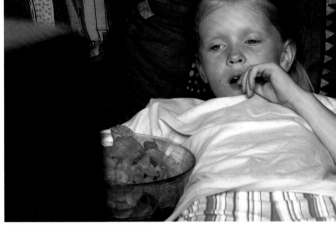

If you spend lots of time watching television and snacking—and not much time running around playing—you are more likely to start gaining weight as you grow older, and you may develop health problems as a result.

What does your gallbladder do? Your gallbladder helps your body digest fat.

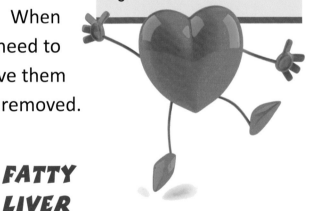

DID YOU KNOW?

Your liver is the largest organ inside your body.

FATTY LIVER

When fat builds up on the liver, it can make your liver swollen. This can cause scarring and permanent liver damage. Your liver is one of the most important parts of your body. It has many jobs, including changing food into energy, cleaning poisons from your blood, and helping with the digestion of your food.

PSEUDOTUMOR CEREBRI

This is a rare cause of very bad headaches that's more common in young people who are obese. Pressure builds up in the brain, as though you had a **tumor**, even though you don't really have a tumor. It causes pain, as well as vomiting, an unsteady way of walking, and vision problems that may become permanent if not treated.

What's a tumor? A tumor is an abnormal growth of cells, forming a mass. A tumor can be malignant (cancerous) or benign (not cancerous).

What is puberty? Puberty is the time when your body goes through a number of physical changes as it becomes an adult body.

POLYCYSTIC OVARY SYNDROME (PCOS)

As they enter **puberty**, girls who are overweight may not get their menstrual periods, because they have too much male hormones in their blood. Although it is normal for girls to have some male hormones in their bodies, too much

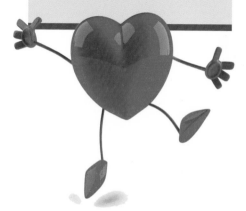

can keep **ovaries** from working normally. It can also make extra hair grow on girls' bodies, and it can make girls have pimples and even go bald. PCOS also goes along with the early stages of type 2 diabetes.

What do ovaries do? Ovaries are the part of a woman's body that make the eggs from which babies can grow. Ovaries also make hormones that help tell a woman's body when to menstruate and how to grow.

DEPRESSION

Everyone feels sad sometimes, but when a person is depressed, she feels sad most of the time, every day. Kids who are overweight and obese are more likely to be depressed. They're also likely to feel bad about themselves. Being depressed can get in the way of a kid being able to do her best at school, at home, and with her friends. It's important to like yourself!

THE GOOD NEWS

If you're overweight or obese, it's never too late to make changes in your life that will help you control your weight. By doing so, you can prevent the health problems that being overweight causes. It's important to do that now, while you're still young—because adults who are overweight and obese are at risk of getting even more diseases.

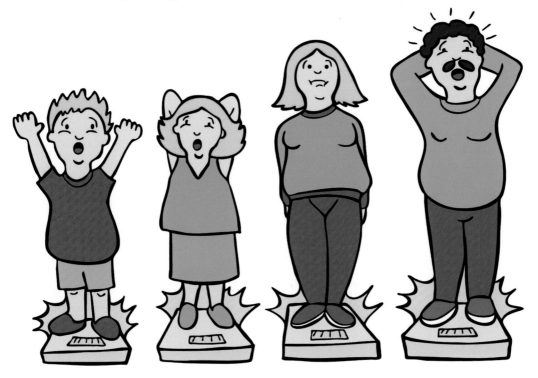

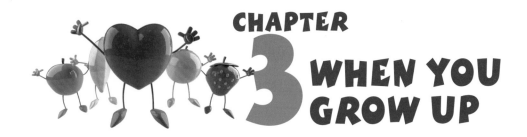

CHAPTER 3
WHEN YOU GROW UP

Adults who are overweight and obese are more likely to get serious illnesses like heart disease, stroke, and cancer.

HEART DISEASE

A person with heart disease often has narrow arteries, because of the buildup of cholesterol inside them. The heart has to work harder, and it may wear out. Angina (chest pain), abnormal heartbeat rhythms, and congestive heart failure (when fluids build up around your heart so it can't do its job well) are all heart conditions that are more likely to happen to people who are overweight and obese. If a person has a heart attack, the flow of blood and oxygen to the heart is interrupted, damaging the heart muscle or stopping it altogether. And you can't live without your heart!

DID YOU KNOW?

Heart disease is the leading cause of death in the United States.

STROKE

During a stroke, blood and oxygen do not flow normally to the brain. Your body's cells need oxygen constantly, and without it, they die. When this happens, parts of your body can stop working and become paralyzed. Sometimes, parts of your brain will no longer work the way they used to. A person may not be able to talk normally, or he may not be able to remember. If a stroke is bad enough, it can also kill a person.

DID YOU KNOW?

Stroke is the third leading cause of death in the United States.

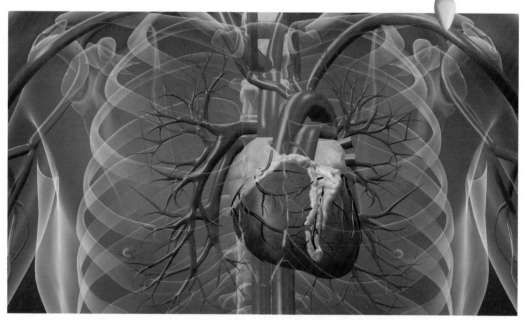

When fat builds up around your heart or inside your blood vessels, it makes your heart have to work harder to move the blood around your body. Eventually, this can make your heart start to wear out.

CANCER

Scientists have discovered that adults who are overweight or obese are more likely to get cancer. Cancer is actually a group of many diseases that all have to do with cells. It happens when cells that are not normal grow and spread very fast.

Normal body cells grow and divide into new cells. This is what happens when you grow, or when your body repairs itself after you've been hurt. Healthy cells know when to stop growing, and over time, they also die. That's normal. Otherwise, you would just grow and grow and grow!

DID YOU KNOW?

Cancer is the second leading cause of death in the United States.

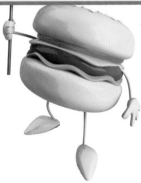

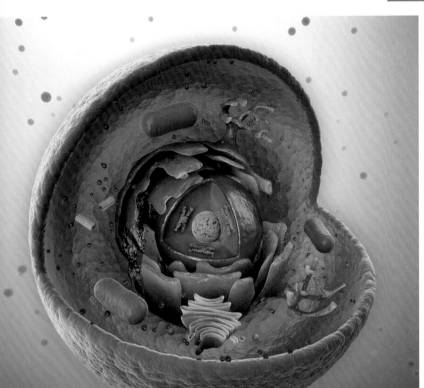

Your body is made up of tiny cells like the one shown here.

Unlike normal, healthy cells, however, cancer cells don't know when to stop growing. They divide over and over again, and they don't die when they should. These unhealthy growths usually clump together to form tumors. The tumor can destroy the normal cells around it and damage the body's other healthy cells. This can make you very sick.

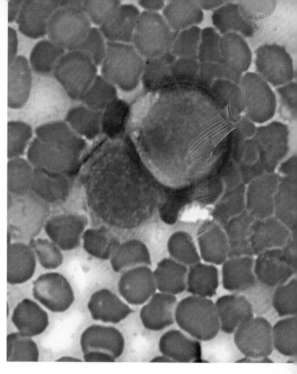

This photo shows cancer cells surrounded by normal, healthy cells.

Sometimes cancer cells break away from the tumor and travel to other areas of the body, where they keep growing and form new tumors. This is how cancer spreads. The spread of a tumor to a new place in the body is called metastasis. When a cancer metastasizes, it is very serious, because it is harder now for doctors to stop its growth.

Doctors aren't sure why some people get cancer and others don't. They do know that cancer is not contagious. You can't catch it from someone else who has it. A germ doesn't cause it, the way germs cause colds or an upset stomach. But certain kinds of things can make you more likely to get cancer, and being overweight is one of these things. Scientists think that fat cells may release hormones that change the way

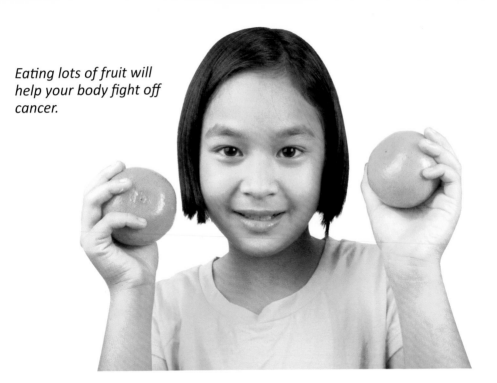

Eating lots of fruit will help your body fight off cancer.

other cells grow, leading to cancer. Also, the kinds of foods that help make a person overweight may also make her more likely to get cancer.

THE GOOD NEWS

Healthy eating and exercise lowers your risk of getting cancer someday. If you lose even 5 to 10 percent of your weight—if you weigh 100 pounds (45 kg), and if that's considered over-weight for your height, that would mean losing just 5 or 10 pounds (2.25 or 4.5 kg)—you can also lower your chances of one day having heart disease or a stroke. Losing weight isn't easy—but it's worth it!

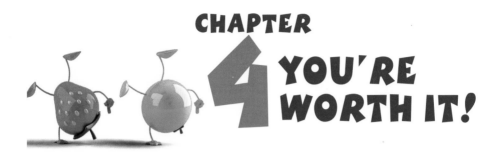

CHAPTER 4
YOU'RE WORTH IT!

Obesity is a big health problem that the entire world is facing. More and more people are overweight than ever before because of changes in our lifestyles—how we eat and move around. The **tendency** to be overweight may also be passed along from parents to their children. So if you're overweight or obese, don't feel like it's your fault. It's a problem that lots of people are facing today.

And it doesn't have any easy answers—not for the world as a whole, and not for individuals. If you or someone you know is overweight or obese, you probably already know how hard it is to lose weight and keep it off. No one should ever be blamed for being overweight. It's a very, very difficult problem.

What does tendency mean? It means the likelihood that something will happen or the likelihood of acting in a certain way.

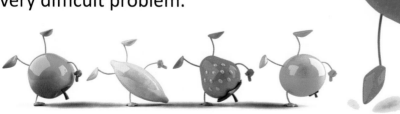

THE FIRST STEP: GET EDUCATED!

The first thing you as an individual can do is to be aware of the problem. Talk about it with your family and friends. The more people know about a problem and the more they think about it and talk about it, the more the world can begin to build healthier ways of living, little by little.

Don't just accept what goes on around you and follow along blindly. Ask questions. Learn about what a healthy lifestyle looks like. Find out about healthier ways to eat. Discover for yourself how exercise helps your body be the best it can be.

DID YOU KNOW?

Scientists have discovered the best combination of foods your body needs to be healthy. A diagram of this combination looks like a pyramid, with the foods you need to eat more at the bottom, and the foods you need to eat less at the top. The U.S. Department of Agriculture, the part of the American government that deals with food, farming, and nutrition, has created a picture called "MyPyramid" to help you understand better how much and what kinds of foods you need to eat in order to be healthy.

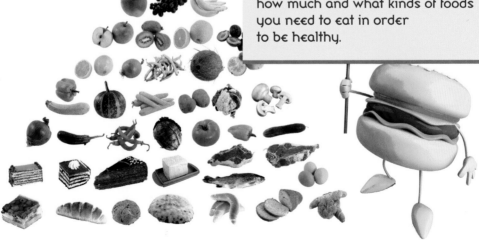

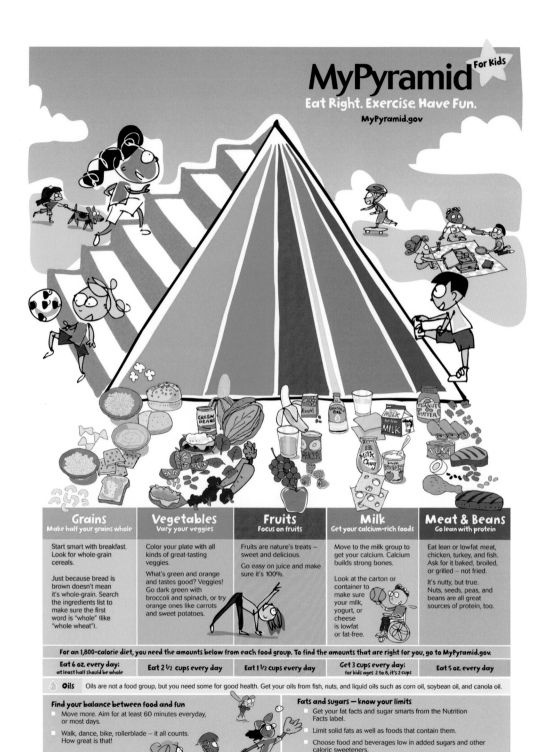

MyPyramid For Kids
Eat Right. Exercise. Have Fun.
MyPyramid.gov

Grains
Make half your grains whole

Start smart with breakfast. Look for whole-grain cereals.

Just because bread is brown doesn't mean it's whole-grain. Search the ingredients list to make sure the first word is "whole" (like "whole wheat").

Vegetables
Vary your veggies

Color your plate with all kinds of great-tasting veggies.

What's green and orange and tastes good? Veggies! Go dark green with broccoli and spinach, or try orange ones like carrots and sweet potatoes.

Fruits
Focus on fruits

Fruits are nature's treats – sweet and delicious.

Go easy on juice and make sure it's 100%.

Milk
Get your calcium-rich foods

Move to the milk group to get your calcium. Calcium builds strong bones.

Look at the carton or container to make sure your milk, yogurt, or cheese is lowfat or fat-free.

Meat & Beans
Go lean with protein

Eat lean or lowfat meat, chicken, turkey, and fish. Ask for it baked, broiled, or grilled – not fried.

It's nutty, but true. Nuts, seeds, peas, and beans are all great sources of protein, too.

For an 1,800-calorie diet, you need the amounts below from each food group. To find the amounts that are right for you, go to MyPyramid.gov.

Grains	Vegetables	Fruits	Milk	Meat & Beans
Eat 6 oz. every day; at least half should be whole	**Eat 2 ½ cups every day**	**Eat 1 ½ cups every day**	**Get 3 cups every day;** for kids ages 2 to 8, it's 2 cups	**Eat 5 oz. every day**

💧 **Oils** Oils are not a food group, but you need some for good health. Get your oils from fish, nuts, and liquid oils such as corn oil, soybean oil, and canola oil.

Find your balance between food and fun
- Move more. Aim for at least 60 minutes everyday, or most days.
- Walk, dance, bike, rollerblade – it all counts. How great is that!

Fats and sugars — know your limits
- Get your fat facts and sugar smarts from the Nutrition Facts label.
- Limit solid fats as well as foods that contain them.
- Choose food and beverages low in added sugars and other caloric sweeteners.

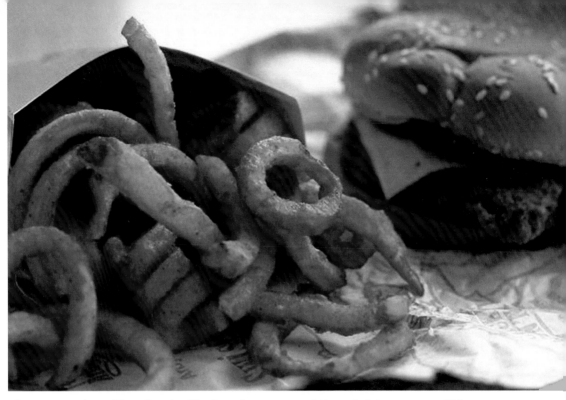

If you eat a lot of fast food—like hamburgers and French fries—you will be more likely to become overweight.

THE SECOND STEP: TAKE AN HONEST LOOK AT YOURSELF!

You may not be overweight or obese now. But as you get older, you might gain weight. To find out if you're likely to have a problem with your weight as you get older, answer the following questions as honestly as you can:

1. Do you usually take less than twenty minutes to eat a meal?
2. After finishing your meal, do you still feel hungry?
3. When you sit down to eat, do you eat everything put in front of you no matter how big the portion size?

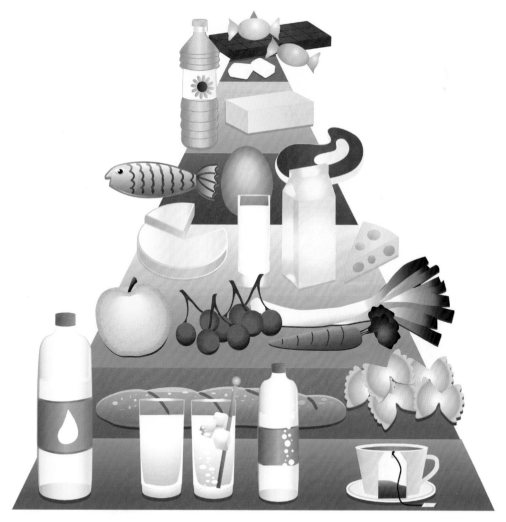

A balanced diet includes the right amounts of different kinds of food. Eating this way is the best way to stay healthy.

4. Does your diet include large amounts of high-sugar or high-fat foods?

5. Do you exercise at least three days each week?

6. Do you eat a balanced diet each and every day?

If you answered yes to the first three questions or no to questions 5 and 6, you may find that you gain weight as you get older. But don't wait till you have a problem! The more weight you have to lose, the harder it is to do. Do what you can to change your lifestyle now.

THE THIRD STEP: TAKE ACTION!

If we're going to lose weight, we need to form new habits. This isn't easy—but new ways of living become easier to do the more we do them. Ask the grownups in your life to help you. (Chances are they need to form new habits too, so you can help each other!) Learn to take care of your body every day.

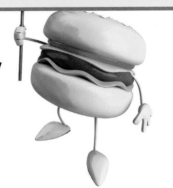

DID YOU KNOW?

Researchers have found that going on a special diet is not usually the best way to lose weight. Diets are just too hard to stick to.

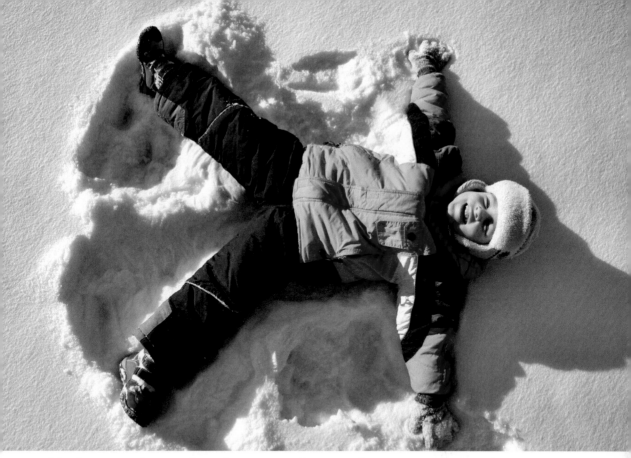

Moving around more doesn't mean you have to play sports or do exercises. It could mean just being outside playing!

Give your body the foods it needs to be healthy. Eating a variety of foods is the best way to get all the vitamins and minerals you need each day, as well as the right balance of carbohydrates, proteins, fats, and calories. Whole or unprocessed foods—foods that are as close as possible to the way they grew naturally, without being frozen, canned, or packaged—are the best choices for getting the nutrients your body needs to stay healthy and grow properly.

Does this mean you have to give up foods like potato chips, candy bars, and cookies forever? No, it's okay to have these foods once in a while. Just don't eat too many of them. To choose health-ier foods, check food labels, and then pick foods that are high in vitamins and min-erals. For example, if you want a snack, an apple or an orange is a **nutritious** choice— but a bag of chips or a candy bar doesn't give you much nutrition, although it does have lots of calories!

What does nutritious mean? Something that's nutritious gives your body the things it needs to be healthy.

When you're eating, pay attention to how your body feels and when your stomach feels full. Sometimes, people eat too much because they don't notice when they need to stop eating. Learn to hear when your body is saying that you've eaten enough.

Your body also needs exercise. If you're already overweight or if you're out of shape, exercise may seem like hard work. You don't have to become an overnight jock—but the more you move around, the more fat you'll burn. Try to spend no more than two hours a day watching television, playing computer games, or doing anything else that means you're sitting down (aside from what you HAVE to do at school). Go for walks, play with

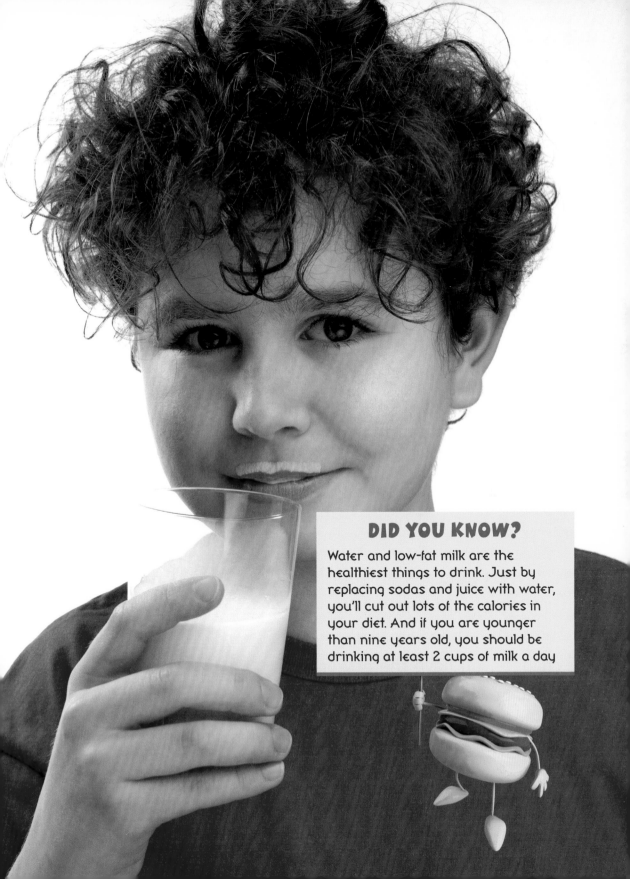

DID YOU KNOW?

Water and low-fat milk are the healthiest things to drink. Just by replacing sodas and juice with water, you'll cut out lots of the calories in your diet. And if you are younger than nine years old, you should be drinking at least 2 cups of milk a day your dog, run up and down stairs. Dance. Jump rope. It doesn't matter WHAT you do, so long as your body is moving.

Learn to take care of your body. Don't try to make your body do without the things it needs, and don't worry about making yourself look like a skinny actor or actress you've seen on television. Instead, feed it when it's hungry. Give it the foods it needs to be healthy. Find fun ways to get more exercise. Get plenty of sleep.

We're all in this together. All of us live in a changing world where eating healthy and exercising have become harder to do. While scientists and doctors search for the answers to this problem, we can do what we can in our individual lives.

And just because you're still a kid doesn't mean you can't begin now. Get educated, be honest with yourself, and take action! No matter how hard it may be to change, you have the power to shape your life. And you're worth it!

DID YOU KNOW?

Exercise should be fun. So pick something you really like to do. You'll be more likely to make it a habit if you like what you're doing. And if you haven't been moving around much lately, start out slowly. Don't overdo it! It will be harder to stick with an exercise program if you make yourself tired and sore at the very beginning.

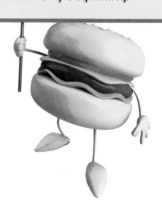

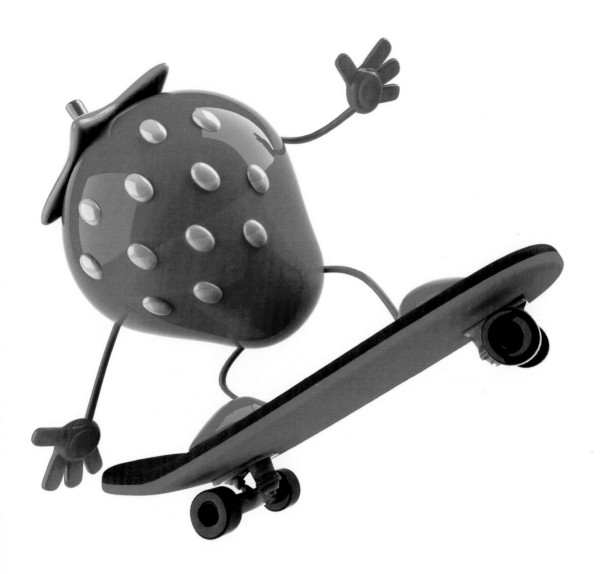

READ MORE ABOUT IT

Bean, Anita. *Awesome Foods for Active Kids: The ABCs of Eating for Energy and Health*. Alameda, Calif.: Hunter House, 2006.

Behan, Eileen. *Fit Kids: Raising Physically and Emotionally Strong Kids with Real Food.* New York: Pocket Publishing, 2001.

Berg, Frances M. *Children and Teens Afraid to Eat.* Hettinger, N.D.: Healthy Weight Network, 2001.

Dolgoff, Joanna. *Red Light, Green Light, Eat Right: The Food Solution That Lets Kids Be Kids.* Emmaus, Penn.: Rodale, 2009.

Gaesser, Glenn. *Big Fat Lies: The Truth About Your Weight and Your Health*. Carlsbad, Calif.: Gürze Books, 2002.

Johnson, Susan, and Laurel Mellin. *Just for Kids! (Obesity Prevention Workbook).* San Anselmo, Calif.: Balboa Publishing, 2002.

Lillien, Lisa. *Hungry Girl 1-2-3: The Easiest, Most Delicious, Guilt-Free Recipes on the Planet.* New York: St. Martin's, 2010.

Vos, Miriam B. *The No-Diet Obesity Solution for Kids*. Bethesda, Md.: AGA Institute, 2009.

Wann, Marilyn. *Fat! So? Because You Don't Have to Apologize for Your Size*. Berkeley. Calif.: Ten Speed Press, 2009.

Zinczenko, David, and Matt Goulding. *Eat This Not That! For Kids!* Emmaus, Penn.: Rodale, 2008.

FIND OUT MORE ON THE INTERNET

Aim for a Healthy Weight: Assess Your Risk
www.nhlbi.nih.gov/health/public/heart/obesity/lose_wt/risk.htm#limitations

American Cancer Society
www.cancer.org

American Obesity Association
www.obesity.org

Children with Diabetes
www.childrenwithdiabetes.com

The Learning Center
www.hebs.scot.nhs.uk/learningcentre/obesity/intro/index.cfm

Move It!
www.fns.usda.gov/tn/tnrockyrun/moveit.htm

MyPyramid Blast Off Game
www.mypyramid.gov/kids/kids_game.html

National Heart, Lung, and Blood Institute (NHLBI)
www.nhlbi.nih.gov

Small Step Kids
www.smallstep.gov/kids/html/games_and_activities.html

The websites listed on this page were active at the time of publication. The publisher is not responsible for websites that have changed their address or discontinued operation since the date of publication. The publisher will review and update the websites upon each reprint.

INDEX

PICTURE CREDITS

ABOUT THE AUTHOR

Helen Thompson lives in upstate New York. She worked first as a social worker and then became a teacher as her second career. She has taught health topics to kids in grades six through eight, and she has attended workshops in nutrition and fitness. Although she has never been an athlete, she enjoys hiking regularly, and works hard to maintain a high-fiber, low-fat diet.

CC

Central Childrens